Soumia Benbernou
Abdelkader Dahmane
Fadila Larbaoui

Anesthesia for obese patients

Soumia Benbernou
Abdelkader Dahmane
Fadila Larbaoui

Anesthesia for obese patients

ScienciaScripts

Cover image: www.ingimage.com

This book is a translation from the original published under ISBN 978-620-6-71126-1.

Publisher:
Sciencia Scripts
is a trademark of
Dodo Books Indian Ocean Ltd. and OmniScriptum S.R.L publishing group

120 High Road, East Finchley, London, N2 9ED, United Kingdom
Str. Armeneasca 28/1, office 1, Chisinau MD-2012, Republic of Moldova, Europe
Printed at: see last page
ISBN: 978-620-7-61658-9

ANAESTHESIA FOR OBESE PATIENTS

PREPARED BY : BENBERNOU SOURNIA, DAHMANE ABDELKADER, BOURADA HORIYA LARBAOUD FADILA, GHOMARD NABIL

TABLE OF CONTENTS

INTRODUCTION

Introduction :

In recent years, obesity has become the number one non-communicable disease in history. Obesity has risen sharply worldwide, including in developing countries. Obesity is a major risk factor for cardiovascular disease, diabetes and cancer, and can put pressure on the healthcare system.
According to recent WHO global estimates:

In 2016, more than 1.9 billion adults were overweight. Of these, more than 650 million were obese.
Overall, around 13% of the world's adult population (11% of men and 15% of women) were obese in 2016.
In Algeria, a recent study highlighted the existence of a high prevalence of overweight and obesity in a sample of school-age children in a large Algerian city.
Consequently, this increase in the prevalence of obesity in our society systematically includes an increase in the number of obese patients requiring surgery for various reasons. The management of these patients is special and requires technical resources and knowledge to optimise the results of their therapeutic management.
Unfortunately, excess weight is correlated with high peri-operative morbidity and mortality. Peri-operative mortality is twice as high for patients whose body mass index is greater than 30kg/m2.
Pre-operative assessment of the obese patient is therefore very important, as it enables problems to be detected and the most appropriate anaesthetic technique to be chosen for the planned surgical procedure. This assessment also makes it possible to devise an appropriate analgesic method, and to prevent the occurrence of postoperative complications.
Intra-operatively, a good knowledge of the changes induced by excess weight on the fate of anaesthetic agents will enable the most appropriate anaesthetic protocol to be chosen with discernment and dosage to be adjusted precisely. The same goes for mastering technical procedures, which can be particularly difficult in obese patients. Post-operatively, these patients require optimal care to avoid complications ranging from simple vitamin deficiency to cardiac arrest.

CHAPTER I
GENERAL INFORMATION ON OBESITY

1. EPIDEMIOLOGY :

1.1. Prevalence :

Modern lifestyles have a huge influence on eating habits. In a fast-growing society, eating patterns are disorganised, and there is a marked tendency to over-consume sugar, fat, alcohol and fast food of all kinds.An increase in sedentary lifestyles and a lack of physical exercise are factors that encourage rapid and significant weight gain.The main causes of the low rate of demand for care, despite the constant increase in the rate of obesity, are :

• The cultural context that tolerates overweight, sometimes even tending to value obesity as a sign of wealth and good health.

• The lack of referral of obese patients by doctors, and sometimes even the underestimation of this pathology.

• Some patients' fear of surgery.

• The denial experienced by some patients who do not consider themselves ill and who feel that they do not need treatment.

1.2. Age :

The prevalence of obesity is highest in the 40-59 age group, with an average age of 48.

1.3. Gender :

The prevalence of obesity is higher among women (38.5%) and men (34.5%).

2. STUDY OF OBESITY :

2.1. Definition of obesity :

General definition: Obesity is defined as an excessive accumulation of fat in the body, with harmful consequences for the individual's physical and mental health. In normal cases, body fat represents around 10 to 15% of the total body weight. % of body weight in young men and 20-25% of body weight in young women.

WHO definition: as a very large accumulation of fat in the body, which can damage general health. It represents an advanced form of "overweight", also known as "overweight", a stage in which the harmful effects of adipose tissue on the body are less significant.

2.2. Assessment of obesity :

2.2.1. Ideal weight (IP) :

There are several methods for calculating your ideal weight.

- **According to Broca's index :**

PI (kg) = Height (cm) - 100

- **Lorenz formula:**

Height (cm) - 150

$$PI\ (kg) = Taille\ (cm) - 100 - \frac{Taille\ (cm) - 150}{X}$$

Or X = 4 for men and X = 2.5 for women

- **According to AZZERA:**

PI = Height (cm) - 100 - (Height (cm) - 150 / 4]

2.2.2. Based on body mass index (BMI) :

$$IMC = \frac{Poids\ (kg)}{Taille\ (m)^2}$$

- **An individual is considered to be obese**:

- When its weight exceeds 20% of its IP

- Obesity is said to be morbid when the actual weight is twice the IBP.

- BMI 18.5 to 24, 9 kg / m2 → ideal weight

BMI 25 kg/m2 - 30 kg/m2 → Overweight

- BMI > 30 kg / m2 → obesity

-BMI > 40 kg / m2 → morbid obesity

-BMI >50 kg / m2⟶ super-morbid obesity

2.3. The different types of obesity according to BMI:

Again based on BMI, we can divide obesity into three different categories. Moderate obesity, severe obesity and morbid obesity.

2.4.3. Moderate obesity :

Moderate obesity is defined as a BMI of between 30 and 35 kg/m2. This is considered to be the least serious form of obesity. However, this in no way means that it poses no health risk to the individual. There is still a significant risk of contracting diseases such as high blood pressure or diabetes. What's more, the risk increases depending on a number of factors, including genetics and the environment.

2.4.4. Severe obesity :

After moderate obesity comes severe obesity. This increasingly worrying form is defined by a BMI of between 35 and 40 kg/m2. As you can imagine, the situation worsens and the risk of suffering from the illnesses already mentioned becomes higher and higher.

2.4.5. Morbid or massive obesity :

If no measures are taken to get rid of all those superfluous kilos, the threshold of morbid obesity can be reached. This is the most dangerous form of obesity. The BMI reaches 40 or even 50 kg/m2 and over, after which it is called "massive obesity". At this level, there is no longer any question of risks, because the diseases that used to threaten the subject are now omnipresent and the person's life is in danger. A person suffering from morbid or massive obesity loses an average of 2 to 5 years' life expectancy.
Health professionals also assess the risks to which an obese person is exposed on the basis of the distribution of their body fat. Obesity can be android or gynoid.

2.5. Types of obesity according to morphology :

2.5.1. Android obesity :

This is the storage of fat mass in the upper part of the body (neck, arms, abdomen). The result of this excess is a large belly. It is generally caused by eating too much and **not doing enough sport**. It can also be due to **hormonal disorders** or **genetic diseases**.

This type of obesity is particularly prevalent in men and is associated with an increased risk of diabetes. type II, hypertension and coronary artery disease. The presence of fatty deposits in the cervical region may interfere with intubation.

2.5.2. Gynoid obesity :

This is the storage of fat mass in the lower part of the body, with adipose tissue distributed mainly on the hips, buttocks and thighs. This type predominates in women, particularly before the menopause.

3. Aetiologies :

Obesity can be explained by a number of factors:

- **Nutrition:** is the leading cause of obesity in adults. A poor diet can have very harmful consequences for health. All it takes is too great an imbalance between what we eat and what we expend in energy, and over a long period of time, for our weight to gradually increase. This can be explained by a lack of physical activity on a daily basis and an excessively sedentary lifestyle (computer, television, etc.). In fact, the causes of obesity can also be eating fatty, salty or sweet foods, in large quantities and without respecting mealtimes, can lead to weight gain.
- **Heredity:** if a person has a relative who is obese or overweight, the risk that he or she will become obese increases. A study has shown that 70% of obese people have at least one relative who suffers from obesity.
- **Psychological factors:** in cases of great distress or stress, there is a tendency to compensate by eating, particularly high-calorie comfort foods.
- **The sornrneil rnanque:** French adults (aged 18-55) sleep an average of 7 hours a night during the week. More than a third sleep only 6 hours a night. What's more, half of teenagers sleep less than 8 hours a night, as opposed to the

recommended 8.5 hours/9.15 hours. Several studies have shown a correlation between short sleep times and high BMI. The risk of obesity increases by 60% when you sleep just 5 hours a night. This is explained by a reduction in leptin and an increase in ghrelin (an appetite-stimulating hormone).

🕓 **Ethical factors:** in the United States, for example, populations of African or Mexican origin are more exposed to obesity than populations of African or Mexican origin. of Asian origin.

🕓 **Medical conditions:** certain endocrine diseases (Cushing's, hypothyroidism, etc.) or therapeutic conditions (corticosteroids, antidepressants, antihistamines, etc.) can promote weight gain.

🕓 **Medication:** some treatments can alter your appetite. To avoid gaining weight as a result of drug treatment, it is advisable to pay attention to your diet.

🕓 **Energy balance:** calorie intake, particularly lipid intake, plays a major role in obesity. Alcohol consumption also appears to be a determining factor. Contrary to the generally accepted view, energy expenditure is increased in obese people. Lack of activity is often the consequence, not necessarily the cause, of obesity.

CHAPTER II
PATHOPHYSIOLOGY OF OBESITY

Obesity is a multifactorial disease, involving a number of behavioural, psychological, social, environmental and biological determinants such as genetic, hormonal, metabolic and pharmacological factors, and evolves in several phases.

1.1. Preclinical phase :

Associated with innate predisposition in individuals. Few studies have evaluated the impact of heredity in the development of obesity. In our series, 60% of patients had parental obesity.

1.2. Creation phase :

Weight gain results from an imbalance between energy intake and energy expenditure.
Explained by :

- Bad eating habits.
- Absence of dietary rhythm with extra-prandial food intake
- Staggering of meals with high calorie content towards the end of the day.
- Increase in fat rations.
- Increase in the calorie content of food.
- The emotional component, with tendencies ranging from hyperphagia to eating disorders.
- Lower energy costs
- Reducing work-related expenses.
- Passive transport facilitation.
- Decrease in physical recreation in favour of sedentary activities (television, computer).

1.3. Maintenance phase :

This phase is accompanied by a new energy balance and changes in storage capacity. Adipocytes hypertrophy and/or increase in number. These phenomena are associated with changes in lipogenesis or lipolysis capacity, which explains the high fat storage capacity and excess weight. This phase leads to the stage of constituted obesity, characterised by the appearance of co-morbidities, both metabolic (type 2 diabetes, hypertension, dyslipidaemia, NASH) and mechanical (sleep apnoea, rheumatological disorders, venous insufficiency, lymphoedema). This phase is also marked by weight fluctuations associated with repeated attempts to lose weight, often followed by weight rebounds. These episodes of weight "yo-yoing" have undeniable psychological consequences (loss of self-esteem, eating disorders) and physical consequences (reduction in lean body mass, changes in energy metabolism), ultimately leading to a worsening of the weight. Clinically, the process of adipose inflation becomes chronic and resistance to weight loss sets in (so-called "refractory" obesity). In E. Koceir's series, the most common eating disorder was hyperphagia, as in our series.

Table VIII: Comparison of eating disorders.

Pays	Auteur	Nombre de patients	Trouble du comportement alimentaire le plus fréquent
Algérie	E. Koceir et al	40	Hyperphagie
Maroc	Notre étude	10	Hyperphagie

2. Complications related to the terrain :

A causal link has been established between obesity and numerous complications known as comorbidities. These can be either life-threatening, or a source of significant disability or reduced life expectancy. But the most important is the risk of surgery associated with these comorbidities.

2.1. Cardiovascular complications :

Most obesity-related cardiac pathologies result from cardiovascular adaptation to excess body mass and increased metabolic demand. Hypertension is the complication most frequently found in obese patients, occurring in almost 34.7% of subjects in the Obépi-Roche study, with 3.6 times more cases of treated hypertension in obese patients than in those with a BMI < 25 kg/m2.Obesity is a significantly increased risk factor for hypertension in the case of abdominal obesity. There are many pathophysiological mechanisms that explain the onset of hypertension in obese patients, including insulin resistance and activation of the sympathetic nervous system, but the main mechanism is the increase in adipose tissue, particularly perivisceral adipose tissue, which is the site of synthesis of angiotensinogen, an activator of the renin-angiotensin system that leads to an increase in blood pressure.

2.1.2. Congestive heart failure :

Increased body fat increases the pre-load on the heart, leading to LVH with dilatation, and hypertension increases the post-load on the heart, leading to increased LVH and ultimately heart failure. The respiratory impact of obesity cannot be overlooked. Sleep apnoea syndrome and alveolar hypoventilation are responsible for right heart failure, ultimately leading to congestive heart failure. Several studies have observed an increase in the size of the left atrium, with an increased risk of atrial fibrillation in obese patients.

2.1.3. Coronary heart disease :

Obesity increases the risk of coronary heart disease, independently of other risk factors such as diabetes, hypertension and hypercholesterolaemia. The relative risk of coronary events is 1.9 for subjects with an initial BMI of more than 29 kg/m2 compared with those with an initial BMI of less than 21 kg/m2, taking into account the presence of co-morbidities associated with obesity.

2.1.4. Venous complications :

Mechanically, obesity leads to significant venous stasis and an alteration in the quality of the blood. capillaries, resulting in return circulation disorders, chronic declining oedema, trophic disorders with dermatophytes and an increased risk of erysipelas.

Any situation with a thromboembolic risk justifies thromboprophylaxis in these patients. Additional risk factors for thrombosis are the result of abdominal obesity: elevation of pro-thrombotic markers, reduced fibrinolytic potential and endothelial dysfunction.

2.1.5. Thromboembolic diseases :

Obesity is a major risk factor in the development of venous thromboembolism, due to the increase in factors that promote Virchow's triad:

• Increased venous stasis.

• Proangiogenic factors: alteration of the endothelium by lipid disorders.

• Hypercoagulability: pro-inflammatory state, increased coagulation factors and reduced fibrinolysis.

The frequent delay in diagnosis and the complexity of the terrain mean that venous thromboembolic disease is more serious and more fatal in these patients. The risk of death from pulmonary embolism in obese patients is multiplied by 12, and more than half of patients who die from PE in the postoperative period are morbidly obese.

2.2. Respiratory complications :

As well as dyspnoea, which is very common, obesity has many respiratory complications that need to be investigated.

2.2.1. Obstructive sleep apnoea hypopnoea syndrome (OSAHS) :

SAHOS is a condition characterised by repeated obstruction of the upper airways responsible for episodes of desaturation and numerous nocturnal awakenings. Its definition includes criteria that must be sought before making the diagnosis, which is only accepted if criterion A and/or criterion B in association with criterion C are present:

A	Hyersomnolence diurne
B	Au moins deux des symptômes suivants : ○ Sommeil non récupérateur ○ Étouffements nocturnes ○ Éveils multiples ○ Fatigue ○ Troubles de concentration
C	> 5 événements obstructifs/heure de sommeil en polysomnographie ou polygraphie de ventilation

Polysomnographic recording is the reference examination for documenting abnormal respiratory events occurring during sleep. The results must always be interpreted in the light of the clinical examination data.

Numerous studies have demonstrated the responsibility of OSAHS in increasing cardiovascular risk, the risk of arterial hypertension, coronary heart disease, rhythm disorders and the occurrence of stroke. OSAHS has an impact on carbohydrate metabolism, and is associated with an increase in insulin resistance, contributing to the development of type 2 diabetes.

2.2.2. Obesity-hypoventilation syndrome (OHSS):

This syndrome is defined by the association of obesity and a daytime hypercapnia of 45 mmHg on blood gases, with no other aetiology to explain it. Blood gases may also show a shunt effect in these patients, defined as a sum of PaO2+PCO2<120 mmHg, or alveolar hypoventilation, defined as hypercapnia of 45 mmHg.

2.2.3. Pulmonary arterial hypertension (PAH):

Pulmonary arterial pressure increases in parallel with weight gain. This is due to pulmonary vasoconstriction induced by chronic hypoxia. Left ventricular dysfunction, increased filling pressures and increased cardiac output all contribute to an increase in pulmonary pressures, defined as mean pulmonary artery pressure (mPAP) > 25 mm Hg at rest. Right heart catheterisation is the reference measurement.

2.3. Metabolic complications :

2.3.1 Type 2 diabetes :

The increase in intra-abdominal, hepatic and muscular fat is accompanied by an increase in circulating free fatty acids in the blood. leading to insulin resistance, the result is a reduction in all the phenomena controlled by insulin, the muscular use of glucose, the slowing down of hepatic glucose production and the inhibition of lipolysis. Insulin resistance often progresses to diabetes, which is a frequent complication of obesity, but is not present in all obese people, as not all obese people are insulin resistant. This can be explained by variations i n fat storage capacity between individuals. In fact, the development of 2 requires two conditions: insulin resistance and B cell dysfunction. Both conditions have a family component which reinforces them, independently of the obesity background.

2.3.2. Dyslipidaemia :

Visceral obesity leads to an increase in the plasma concentration o f free fatty acids through the hydrolysis of triglycerides stored in adipose tissue. This increase favours the accumulation of triglycerides in the muscles and liver and promotes insulin resistance. The hyperinsulinaemia generated then activates the expression of genes regulating sterol transport, contributing to dyslipidaemia but also increasing insulin resistance. Hepatic production of VLDL (very low density lipoprotein) and triglycerides is increased. The increased transfer of triglycerides from VLDL to HDL(high density lipoprotein) will cause HDL particles to become unstable. Hypertriglyceridaemia contributes to the formation of dense LDL (low density lipoprotein) particles, which are particularly atherogenic, as are hypertriglyceridaemia and a reduction in HDL.

2.3.3. Metabolic syndrome

A controversial entity, defined by the American Heart Association and the National Heart Lung And Blood Institute. By the combination of three or more of the criteria listed in table X :

Critère	Seuils
Obésité abdominale	≥ 102 cm chez les hommes ≥ 88 cm chez les femmes
Hypertriglycéridémie Faibles taux de cholestérol HDL (un traitement spécifique à ce trouble peut également servir d'indicateur)	≥ 1,7 mmol/L < 1,0 mmol/L chez les hommes < 1,3 mmol/L chez les femmes
Hypertension (un traitement antihypertenseur chez un patient avec des antécédents d'hypertension peut également servir d'indicateur)	Tension systolique ≥ 130 mmHg Ou Tension diastolique ≥ 85 mmHg
Glycémie à jeun élevée (un traitement antidiabétique peut également servir d'indicateur)	≥ 5,5 mmol/L

Other biological abnormalities are also common in obese subjects: hyperuricaemia often associated with hypertriglyceridaemia, coagulation abnormalities and fibrinolysis with a high risk of venous thrombosis.

2.4. Endocrine repercussions :

Obesity has multiple effects on female reproduction, starting at an early age. The risk of precocious puberty is higher i n obese girls. Later in life, obesity is responsible for a reduction in fertility, with a high risk of anovulation either through central hypogonadism or by aggravating the underlying polycystic ovary syndrome. Obesity is present in 30-75% of cases of polycystic ovary syndrome

(PCOS). The influence of obesity on the expression of PCOS is complex, with areas of uncertainty, but obesity unambiguously influences the development of hyperandrogenism by a number of mechanisms: compensatory hyperinsulinaemia for insulin resistance, a reduction in SHBG (sex hormone banding globulin) responsible for an increase in the free fraction of androgens, unidentified intrauterine factors, and a direct effect of leptin on ovarian function. The PCOS phenotype of obese women is marked by greater hyperandrogenism, a high prevalence of metabolic abnormalities influenced by obesity, more menstrual cycle abnormalities and a reduced response to ovulation-inducing treatment. In men, the impact of obesity on spontaneous fertility has been less studied than in women. However, a hormonal profile associating hypogonadotropic hypogonadism, hyperestrogenism and a decrease in SHBG has been described, at To date, several epidemiological studies have associated male obesity with hypofertility in couples.

2.5. Gastrointestinal disorders :

Biliary lithiasis, hepatic steatosis and gastro-oesophageal reflux disease (GERD) are the most frequently encountered disorders of the digestive system.

2.5.1. Hepatic steatosis :

Non-alcoholic steatohepatitis is one of the least recognised complications of obesity, metabolic syndrome and type 2 diabetes. Anatomically defined as an accumulation of triglycerides in the hepatocytes, it differs from common steatosis in having an inflammatory infiltration and a fibrosing evolution independent of alcohol consumption, which can lead to genuine cirrhosis and be a starting point for hepatocellular carcinoma. The diagnosis is suggested by the presence of steatotic hepatomegaly (on ultrasound), or a moderate increase in liver enzymes, but can only be confirmed by liver biopsy. Lesions vary in intensity but typically include steatosis, inflammation, hyalinosis with Mallory bodies and fibrosis. The progression from fibrosis to cirrhosis is unpredictable. Weight reduction and the use of insulin-sensitising agents such as metformin or thiazolidine-diones improve steatosis and inflammation, confirming the role of obesity and insulin resistance.

2.5.2. GERD :

Gastro-oesophageal reflux is twice as common in obese people and helps to explain the increased risk of oesophageal adenocarcinoma observed in obese subjects.

2.5.3. Biliary lithiasis :

The annual incidence of silent biliary lithiasis is multiplied by 7 in obese women. The lithogenic index of bile is correlated with BMI. Furthermore, rapid weight loss following bariatric surgery or a low-calorie diet increases the risk of lithiasis by significantly reducing vesicular emptying.

2.6. Renal complications :

Renal failure is one of the pathologies associated with obesity, as demonstrated by numerous epidemiological studies. These include segmental and focal glomerulosclerosis or isolated glomerulomegaly, the prevalence of which increases by a factor of 10 in the case of massive or central obesity. Obesity is also an aggravating factor in other types of kidney disease, such as IgA nephropathy (Berger's disease), which progresses more rapidly to chronic renal failure. Finally, obesity is a risk factor for urinary lithiasis. The mechanisms involved are still not fully understood. The role of co-morbidities (hypertension, type 2 diabetes, dyslipidaemia) is predominant, but it cannot be ruled out that obesity has a direct effect via the secretion of adipokines.Experimental data indicate that excess leptin and resistin and reduced adipokine have a deleterious effect on renal function. Microalbuminuria is one of the first markers of obesity-related nephropathy.

2.7. Cancers :

A systematic review and meta-analysis of prospective observational studies involving almost 300,000 incident cases showed that an increase in body weight of 5kg/m2 increases the relative risk of cancers of the oesophagus, bile ducts, kidneys, breast and endometrium in women, and of colon, kidney and thyroid cancers in men. Other cancers - ovarian, pancreatic and liver - would also be favoured by obesity.The RR of breast cancer mortality increases proportionally with the degree of excess weight, rising from 1 for a BMI < 25, to 1.34 in the case of overweight, 1.63 in the case of obesity and 2.12 in the case of massive obesity. Excess lipid intake and increased oestradiolaemia are thought to be responsible for the excess breast cancer in obese women.

2.8. Osteoarticular complications :

The repercussions of obesity on the osteoarticular system are frequent and linked to the mechanical stresses exerted on the cartilage of the main weight-bearing joints - the knees, hips and lumbar spine. The result is an increased sedentary lifestyle, which contributes to obesity, and disability, often leading to occupational invalidity. Gonarthrosis occurs in 50% of women with massive obesity. In a British cohort, BMI was associated with a relative risk of prosthetic knee replacement of 10.5 compared with 2.5 for the hip. Obesity aggravates congenital hip malformations. It is also a factor in osteonecrosis of the femoral head in men. Obesity is still associated with a high prevalence of lumbar degenerative disc disease, ankle tendonitis and plantar fasciitis.

2.9. Dermatological complications :

Certain benign dermatoses are more common in obese people:

• Mycosis of the folds, intertrigo or involvement of the large folds (submammary, axillae, abdominal folds, inguinal folds, intergluteal folds), due to maceration.

• Acne caused by an increase in androgen hormones.

• Cellulite, which is a superficial lipodystrophy combining adipose tissue, oedema and fibrosis in the adipocytes, and which can be seen in slim people.

• Hyperhidrosis (or excessive sweating).

• Stretch marks, which can appear when there is a great deal of tension on the skin, such as major weight gain or pregnancy.

• Acanthosis nigricans, a hyperpigmentation and thickening of the large folds, is a dermatosis specific to obesity, and should be investigated for deep neoplasia if it appears in a non-obese subject.

• Molluscum pendulum are benign pedunculated skin growths.

• Plantar hyperkeratosis, encouraged by excess weight through mechanical action.

2.1 O. Psychological repercussions :

Massive obesity undeniably diminishes quality of life and stigmatises people in today's socio-cultural environment, which, while encouraging obesity, has a negative prejudice against it. The prevailing 'thin' ideal contributes to the development of a feeling of malaise and exclusion, which risks reinforcing existing eating disorders and leading to a depressive syndrome. However, obesity can also be a form of defence and adaptation to personal problems, creating an apparent balance that can be destabilised after weight loss, leading to depressive decompensation.

2.1.1. Mortality :

According to the WHO, the relationship between mortality and BMI follows an ascending curve: as BMI increases, so does the relative risk of death, reaching 1.5 for a BMI of between 25 and 30. Above a BMI of 30, the risk of death rises more rapidly, quickly reaching 2.5 for a BMI of 35. Obesity reduces life expectancy at the age of 40 by 7.1 years in women and 5.8 years in non-smoking men.

3. PHARMACOLOGICAL CHANGES IN OBESE SUBJECTS :

A good understanding of the changes induced by obesity in the fate of anaesthetic agents means that the most appropriate anaesthetic protocol can be chosen with discernment, and dosages adjusted precisely. The main changes induced by obesity are pharmacokinetic, affecting the absorption, distribution and elimination of drugs.

3.1.Pharmacokinetic changes :

3.1.1. Absorption :

Obesity in itself does not affect the digestive absorption of anaesthetic agents. However, some bariatric surgery procedures are likely to induce malabsorption syndromes.

3.1.2. Distribution: Binding to plasma proteins: In the context of the inflammatory syndrome associated with obesity, concentrations of acid a1glycoprotein may be doubled in obese subjects compared with those in normal subjects. observed in subjects of normal weight. There is then a reduction in the free, active fraction of weakly basic agents which bind to this protein, such as erythromycin, lidocaine, bupivacaine, propranolol, alfentanil, fentanyl (in part), sufentanil, remifentanil or verapamil, for example.

3.1.3. Distribution volumes :

Changes in volumes of distribution induced by obesity are multifactorial. One of the main factors is the increase in body fat. Obesity is also accompanied by an increase in blood volume and in the size of the main organs, which can lead to an increase in the volume of the central compartment. Lean body mass is also increased.The increase in the equilibrium volume of distribution of a given compound depends on the relative affinity of the compound for different tissues. The distribution of water-soluble agents, whose volumes of distribution are often smaller than those of liposoluble agents, is generally only slightly altered. The distribution of agents in adipose tissue depends on their liposolubility, which is most often expressed by the octanol/water partition coefficient P, although this parameter may not be reliable. not always be a very good reflection of in-vivo liposolubility. Some agents have a P coefficient that reflects a good affinity for lipids and the ability to cross lipid barriers without this coefficient allowing them to be distributed extensively in adipose tissue. This is the case with propofol, which has a P value of less than 20. The volume of distribution at equilibrium (V.ss) will be increased in obese patients, but the increase will be proportional to the increase in body weight. Other agents distribute preferentially in adipose tissue, such as midazolam (P=34), thiopental (P=89) and diazepam (P=309). In this case, the increase in s.v. will be proportionally greater than the increase in body weight.

3.1.4. Elimination by hepatic metabolism :

Obesity is associated with an increase in cardiac output, blood volume and splanchnic output, although there is no direct evidence of an increase in hepatic blood flow; for example, the clearance of lidocaine, an agent with a high hepatic extraction coefficient, whose systemic clearance is close to functional hepatic blood flow, is not increased by obesity. The livers of obese subjects are larger than those of normal-weight subjects, due to an increase in the number and size of parenchymal cells. However, obesity leads to fatty infiltration of the liver, and even hepatic fibrosis, which can compromise the functioning of this organ even though the usual liver function tests are normal. The clearance of most agents undergoing phase I metabolism (oxidation, reduction, hydrolysis) is little altered in obese subjects, as is that of acetylated agents, despite increased activity of certain P450 cytochromes. On the other hand, hepatic clearance of conjugated agents increases in a way that is closely correlated with the increase in body weight.

3.1.5. Renal elimination :

The size of the kidneys, like that of most other organs, is increased in the obese. Glomerular filtration rate and tubular secretion are increased in the obese. Consequently, the clearance of agents eliminated by glomerular filtration is increased in the obese.

3.2. Choice of anaesthetic agents :

The study of obesity-induced changes in the fate of anaesthetic agents shows that it is impossible to have a clear-cut, unambiguous attitude, and that the therapeutic regimen must be developed on a case-by-case basis, taking into account the known characteristics of the agent itself and not just the pharmacological class to which it belongs.

3.2.1. Intravenous hypnotics :

3.2.1.1. Thiopental :

Thiopental is a highly lipid-soluble agent. This property results in an increased equilibrium volume of distribution in obese patients. As a result, although elimination clearance is high in obese patients, thiopental elimination is delayed in this population (28h versus 6.3h in the control group), so it does not seem ideal to propose thiopental as an anaesthetic induction agent in obese patients, especially when the proposed surgical technique is of short duration. If this is not the case, appropriate doses of thiopental should be proposed for obese patients. As early as 1969, some authors argued that the dose of thiopental could be determined on the basis of lean body mass. This can be calculated using the following formula:

- For men: 1.1 x weight - 128 x (weight/height) 2
- For women: 1.07 x weight - 148 x (weight/height) 2
- SFAR 2012: 3-5 mg/Kg of actual weight.
- JARCA 2006: 7.5 mg/Kg ideal weight.

From a practical point of view, Buckley et al. recommended the administration of a dose higher than 7.5 mg/kg for induction on the basis of ideal weight. The need for this higher dose was based on the increased cardiac output frequently seen in morbidly obese patients, resulting in lower plasma concentrations.

3.2.1.2. Propofol :

The octanol/water partition coefficient of propofol shows that it is a fat-soluble agent, but not sufficiently so to concentrate preferentially in adipose tissue. Its equilibrium volume of distribution therefore increases in proportion to body weight. Elimination clearance of propofol also increases with body weight. Consequently, the opposing influences of these two changes on the elimination half-life cancel each other out, and this parameter is not particularly prolonged in obese patients. The dose of propofol used for anaesthetic induction can be calculated on the basis of weight. When obese patients are anaesthetised with propofol on the basis of their total weight, anaesthesia can be deep and the haemodynamic consequences can be harmful. For the maintenance of anaesthesia, propofol doses must therefore be adjusted to actual weight. In AIVOC, the Marsh model (which takes real weight into account) can be used in obese subjects.

Recommended dosage :

- SFAR 2012: 2-3 mg/Kg of actual weight.
- MAPAR 2010: ideal weight + 0.4 times overweight.

3.2.1.3. Benzodiazepines :

The distribution of benzodiazepines in adipose tissue depends on their liposolubility. Midazolam and diazepam are preferentially stored in fat and therefore tend to accumulate in obese patients. These products are also metabolised by oxidation, and their clearance is not increased in obese patients. Their use in bariatric surgery is therefore not recommended.

3.2.1.4. Ketamine :

There are no data on the pharmacology of ketamine in obese patients. Some authors recommend its use in small doses for short procedures with spontaneous ventilation because of its low impact on cardiorespiratory functions and its usefulness in postoperative analgesia.

3.2.1.5. Inhaled agents :

Fat-soluble halogenated anaesthetics tend to accumulate in adipose tissue and the quantity administered increases with body weight for the same pharmacological effect. In obese patients, this can lead to delayed awakenings. In clinical studies, awakening occurred more rapidly with sevoflurane or desflurane than with propofol or isoflurane. La colla et al compared the pharmacokinetics of desflurane and sevoflurane in two groups of morbidly obese patients. The results showed that the F(A)/F(I) ratio (alveolar fraction/inhaled fraction) was significantly greater in the desflurane group, with desflurane being eliminated more rapidly, enabling the patient to wake up and regain protective airway reflexes sooner. The study by M.C. Vallejo et al did not find any notable advantages for desflurane over sevoflurane, although both have been identified as the molecules of choice in obese subjects. As for nitrous oxide, its use is very limited in bariatric surgery, due to the intestinal distension it causes, which complicates the surgery.

3.2.2. Morphinomimetics :

The pharmacokinetics of fentanyl and alfentanyl have been little studied in obese patients. Despite the liposolubility of fentanyl, its distribution is not particularly high in obese patients. It is therefore advisable to use it in relation to the ideal weight. Sufentanyl, which has an octanol/water partition coefficient of 1754, has an increased volume of distribution in obese patients. However, this increase has no significant impact on its metabolism. The morphinomimetic which currently offers the most advantages for anaesthesia of the obese seems to be remifentanyl, although it is not widely available. This is easily explained by its pharmacological properties: small volume of distribution, high clearance, absence of residual effects, particularly respiratory effects. It should be prescribed according to the usual regimens and depending on ideal weight.

3.2.3. Muscle relaxants :

Being water-soluble, non-depolarising curares do not show a significant increase in their volume of distribution. In order to limit an increase in the duration of neuromuscular block, muscle relaxants should be administered on the basis of ideal body weight. When 0.1mg/kg vecuronium is administered to obese subjects, a delayed decurarisation is observed compared with the control group. This delay in decurarisation is attributable to the relative overdose induced by the administration of vecuronium in relation to the total weight of the obese subject, even though its kinetics are little altered because it is water-soluble. Curares of this type, which also include recuronium,atracurium and cisatracurium should be administered on the basis of ideal body weight. As far as depolarising curares are concerned, it should be remembered that the activity of plasma pseudo cholinesterases increases with body mass index. This is likely to increase the need for succinylcholine without altering the duration of action of this agent. Succinylcholine should therefore, be administered on the basis of total weight. This analysis can be extended to mivacurium without being definitive. A study comparing the use of mivacurium on the basis of total weight in morbidly obese and non-obese patients found no significant difference between the two study groups. However, other studies recommend using doses of mivacurium based on ideal weight in cases of obesity.

CHAPTER III
ANAESTHETIC MANAGEMENT OF THE OBESE PATIENT

1. Pre-operative period :

1.1. Anaesthetic consultation :

Prior to any anaesthesia, the patient and the anaesthetist/resuscitation doctor and the anaesthetist/resuscitation medical assistant meet to exchange information, assess the patient's state of health and formulate the anaesthetic strategy. The purpose of examining the obese patient in the anaesthetic consultation is to understand the co-morbidities associated with obesity that may interfere with perioperative management, and also to inform the patient about the anaesthetic technique and any complications that may arise during the perioperative period, and the measures taken to limit them.

1.1.1. Questioning :

- Morphological data: age; weight, height, sex.
- BMI calculation: **weight [kg] / height [rn]^2**
- Questioning: to find out about the patient's personal medical and surgical history, as well as any family history.
- Calculation of ideal theoretical weight and adjusted weight.
- any allergies or atopic conditions.
- toxic habits: tobacco; alcohol; drug addiction.
- The presence of snoring, episodes of nocturnal apnoea, frequent awakenings during sleep (e.g. vocalisation, changes in position, movements of the extremities), morning headaches and daytime drowsiness will suggest OSA.
- **The** search for **obesity hypoventilation syndrome**:

✓ chronic alveolar hypoventilation $PaCO_2 > 45$ mm Hg $PaO_2 < 70$ mm Hg
✓ obesity (BMI > 30 kg/m2)

✓ the absence of associated respiratory disease - regardless of whether or not it is associated with OSA.

1.1.2. Examination of the upper airways :

Obesity is a risk factor for difficult ventilation and intubation. The clinical examination must be particularly careful, looking for other factors predictive of intubation and difficult ventilation.

✓ **Predictive criteria for ventilation in a difficult rnasque :**

- age > 55
- body mass index BMI > 26 kg/m2
- edentulism
- snoring
- beard
- OSA
- Limiting mandibular protrusion

The presence of two factors is predictive of difficult mask ventilation. A thyro-chin distance of less than 6.5cm combined with snoring are predictive criteria of impossible ventilation.In the obese, cervical mobility is often limited by the chin and thoracic fat at the front and cervical fat at the back, often associated with cervical osteoarthritis. The larynx is generally high and anterior.

✓ **Predictive criteria for difficult intubation :**

- BMI >35
- mouth opening <3.5 cm and dental condition
- Macroglossia
- short neck
- thyromental distance < 6.5cm (see appendix 1)
- Mallampati classes 3 and 4 (see appendix 2)
- Cormack score 2b and 3a direct laryngoscopy (see appendix 3)
- History of difficult intubation
- OSA and neck circumference >60cm
- Cervico-facial pathology, burns

• Pre-eclampsia

1.1.3. Assessment of respiratory function :

Respiratory complications are the leading cause of peri-morbidity. in obese patients. Preoperative respiratory assessment is an important step in their prevention.When questioning the patient, it is important to look for symptoms suggestive of obesity-related respiratory pathology: obesity hypoventilation syndrome, sleep apnoea syndrome, episodes of upper airway obstruction or associated respiratory insufficiency. As well as a thoracic deformity that may lead to respiratory dysfunction. Preoperative preparation using respiratory physiotherapy may be indicated, particularly in patients with COPD. Obstructive sleep apnoea syndrome (OSA) should be systematically considered in the presence of morbid obesity. The search is carried out by questioning the patient and spouse using the **"STOP!BANG"** questionnaire: a score of **3 points** or more should prompt a polysomnographic recording; if positive, the patient should be fitted with an appliance (see appendix 4). Patients fitted with ventilation devices should bring their devices with them when they are admitted to hospital, so that they can resume night-time positive pressure ventilation on the first postoperative night.

1.1.4. Cardiovascular assessment :

Coronary artery disease is the second leading cause of post-operative mortality in obese patients, so it is important to screen for subclinical coronary artery disease and to look for stress symptoms. The NYHA score is calculated to assess cardiac risk in the context of surgery, as is the Lee score in patients with coronary artery disease (see appendices 5-6). There is also an assessment of the risk of thromboembolic disease, which is a frequent post-operative complication in obese patients and increases with BMI.

1.1.5. Digestive and metabolic assessment :

Obese patients have reduced gastric emptying, which is why they are considered to have a full stomach; excess weight, in particular the increase in abdominal circumference, increases intra-abdominal pressure and reduces lower sphincter pressure, which increases the risk of inhalation. These physiological and anatomical changes can lead to GERD, which exposes the obese patient to an increased risk of inhalation. Assess the risk of postoperative nausea and vomiting (PONV) using the simplified **Apfel score** (see appendix 7).Obesity is often associated with glucose intolerance and type II diabetes, and it is important to ensure that the latter is balanced before the operation and to assess its repercussions. For the pre-operative fasting period, a delay of 2 hours is required for clear liquids, 6 hours for a light meal and at least 8 hours for a full meal.

1.2.6. Assessment of venous capital :

Venous access in obese patients can be difficult due to the importance of the adipose layer, which makes the veins deep and invisible to the surgeon. To facilitate vascular access, ultrasound can be used as an aid. When venous access is very difficult or impossible and the operation requires it, a central venous catheter may need to be inserted preoperatively.

1.1.7. Paraclinical examinations :

The request for standard complementary examinations depends on the medical pathology, the type of surgery and the conditions of care. There is no consensus on this, apart from the grouping card, which must be systematically required for all surgical procedures.-ECG according to age and sex: men > 45 years and women > 50 years, apart from severely obese patients BMI >40 and patients at risk of coronary artery disease. Other specific examinations adapted to co-morbidities. :

EFR, cardiac ultrasound, stress test, cardiac scintigraphy, coronography.
- Polysomnography, requested in cases of suspected OSA.

1.1.8. Assessment of surgical risk factors :

The ASA score: Indicator of overall perioperative mortality used by the American Society of Anesthesiologists, which classifies patients into 6 categories:

- **ASA 1:** Normal patient
- **ASA 2:** Patient with moderate systemic abnormality.
- **ASA 3:** Patient with severe systemic abnormality.
- **ASA 4:** Patient with severe systemic abnormality representing a constant threat to life.
- **ASA 5:** Moribund patient unlikely to survive without surgery.
- **ASA 6:** Patient declared brain dead whose organs are removed for

transplantation.

1.1.9. Choice of anaesthetic technique :

Locoregional anaesthesia is preferred, as it reduces the risks associated with difficult intubation, inhalation and the accumulation of intravenous anaesthetic agents. If a general anaesthetic is required, it is best performed in the presence of two anaesthetists.

1.2. Anaesthetic requirements :

❖ Preoperative weight loss is recommended to reduce intraoperative complications.

❖ Smoking cessation should be encouraged preoperatively to minimise the respiratory risk.

❖ Ensure that the equipment is appropriate for the patient's weight:

· Operating table with a capacity > 160 kg.

· A blood pressure cuff one and a half times the circumference of the arm

· Particular care must be taken to protect the support points with agar-type materials.

· Difficult installation requires a large number of staff.

· The use of lateral sliding transfer devices to move obese patients.

❖ ALR should be preferred wherever possible.

❖ Prevention of nausea and vomiting.

❖ Ensure adequate pre-oxygenation.

❖ Plan a strategy for intubation and difficult ventilation.

❖ Antibiotic prophylaxis adapted to adjusted or ideal weight

❖ Systematic monitoring of temperature, depth of anaesthesia and curarisation.

❖ The use of anaesthetic drugs that are the least liposoluble, rapidly reversible, short-acting and with a rapid onset of action.

❖ Titration of anaesthetic agents.

❖ Ensuring optimal haematosis through alveolar recruitment.

❖ Ensure multimodal analgesia with doses adjusted to ideal weight.

❖ Prevention of thromboembolic disease.

❖ prevent the risk of hypothermia by actively warming up.

1.3. Inform the patient :

In the same way as for the pre-anaesthetic questionnaire, written information concerning anaesthesia and transfusion can be given to the patient before the pre-anaesthetic consultation. This method usually allows the patient to read the information carefully and, if necessary, to ask the anaesthetist for further details during the consultation. Experience shows that patients also ask questions about the procedure. It is the anaesthetist's responsibility to explain the planned procedure to the patient or to give him or her information about it.

2. Intraoperative management :

2.1. Preparing the patient :

2.1.1. Prevention of thromboembolic disease :

As the risk of VTE is particularly high in obese patients, it can be prevented by using intermittent external pneumatic compression stockings of the lower limbs peroperatively, and continuing postoperatively in association with low molecular weight heparin in preventive doses adapted to the patient's weight (see appendix 8).

2.1.2. Placement of a venous line :

Inserting a peripheral venous line may prove difficult - the value of ultrasound location or inserting a central catheter.

2.1.3. Premedication :

Intramuscular or subcutaneous premedication should be avoided because of the unpredictability of drug absorption by adipose tissue. In patients with OSA, premedication with benzodiazepines is formally contraindicated. It may induce apnoea, and a single dose of intramuscular Midazolam (0.08 mg kg-1) has been shown to increase the risk of desaturation. The use of metoclopramide to increase the tone of the gastro-oesophageal sphincter and reduce the risk of inhalation In patients with GERD, H2 blockers should be administered prior to surgery to reduce the volume of gastric contents and increase their pH.

2.1.4. Antibiotic prophylaxis :

The latest SFAR 2018 recommendations on perioperative antibiotic prophylaxis have clearly defined antibiotic prophylaxis for obese patients. In obese patients (patients weighing more than 100 kg and body mass index > 35kg/m2), betalactam doses should be double those recommended for non-obese patients. For vancocymine and gentamicin, antibiotic prophylaxis doses are calculated on the basis of actual weight.

2.2 Installation and monitoring :

2.2.1. Installation on the operating table :

✓ Standard operating tables can support weights of up to 130-160 kg. Beyond that, there are specialised tables for weights of up to 450 kg, with a wider, better padded top.
✓ Moving the patient often requires the cooperation of all the OR staff.
✓ The support points are protected before induction and checked regularly to prevent peripheral vascular and nerve compression.
✓ Lateral sliding transfer devices make moving the patient much easier.
✓ Supine proclivity with the head elevated: this is the position of choice for obese patients at induction or intraoperatively. It limits thoracic compression by the abdominal visceral mass.
✓ The sitting or semi-seated position poses few respiratory problems, with little change in the ventilation/perfusion ratio.
✓ Haemodynamics. The lateral decubitus position is often preferred, with a reservation about the right lateral decubitus position, where the vena cava syndrome is often significant.
✓ The Trendelenburg position: is the most deleterious from the respiratory point of view. In addition to the difficulty in expanding the lungs, which may be greater in laparoscopy, the risk of atelectasis and the likelihood of selective intubation is high.

2.2.2. Hemodynamic monitoring :

Haemodynamic monitoring of the obese patient is not specific, but it is vital that it is adapted to the patient's morphology and history.

2.2.3. A standard electrocardioscope has five parameters:

Non-invasive blood pressure, heart rate, respiratory rate, peripheral measurement of pulsed oxygen saturation (SPO2). ECG scope.

2.2.4. Non-invasive measurement of blood pressure :

This should be done with a cuff of the correct size (1.5 times the circumference of the arm). Figures obtained with a cuff that is too small will overestimate blood pressure.

✓ Capnography

✓ Curarisation monitoring essential.

✓ Monitoring the depth of anaesthesia (the bi-spectral index)

✓ Temperature monitoring

✓ Capillary glycaemia is based on the patient's history.

2.3. Pre-oxygenation :

The risk of rapid desaturation (decrease in functional residual capacity and increase in oxygen consumption), difficult mask ventilation or difficult intubation make induction a high-risk period for obese patients. Pre-oxygenation in the procline position delays desaturation in obese patients, with a gain of almost one minute compared with strict decubitus Applying a PEEP (positive expiratory pressure) of at least 10 cmH2O in CPAP mode during pre-oxygenation and for 5 minutes after induction reduces post-intubation atelectasis. Maintaining PEEP would improve PaO2 and increase apnoea time by approximately one minute. Non-invasive ventilation (NIV) in inspiratory aid (IA) + PEEP mode for 5 minutes would also improve preoxygenation in terms of efficiency and prevention of desaturation. The combination of non-invasive ventilation immediately followed by a recruitment manoeuvre seems to be the ideal proposal.

2.6. Anaesthetic induction in obese patients :

Induction must be carried out by at least two anaesthetists, one of whom must be experienced.

2.4.1. The choice of drugs : 1- Thiopental :

As with other highly lipophilic drugs, the terminal and steady-state volumes of distribution of thiopental are three to four times higher in obese patients, so a prolonged effect of this drug will be expected. Extensive research into significant respiratory events in the recovery room has separately identified obesity and thiopental use as risk factors for postoperative hypoxaemia. Under these conditions, it may not be ideal to propose thiopental as an induction agent for anaesthesia in obese patients, especially for procedures of relatively short duration.

2- Propofol :

Propofol is certainly a fat-soluble agent; there is no accumulation when a dose comparable to that proposed for subjects of normal weight is used. Propofol is eliminated after being conjugated: its elimination clearance also increases with body weight. The dose should be calculated on the basis of the adjusted weight, ideally titrated with AIVOC.

3- Etomidate :

There are no studies in obese patients. It is also a fat-soluble molecule, and given that there is a probable increase in the volume of distribution, the induction dose should be based on total weight.

4- Ketamine :

Ketamine is a highly lipid-soluble agent, so the volume of distribution could theoretically be increased in obese patients, with a risk of accumulation.

5- Benzodiazepines :

Their wide distribution in fat and long elimination half-life explain their prolonged effects, which should be avoided.

6- Curares :

Curares are water-soluble agents. The increase in the body's water compartments in obese patients explains the difficulties encountered in specifying dosage regimens for this population.

· **For suxarnethoniurn**: Due to an increase in pseudocholinesterase activity in obese patients, the dosage of succinylcholine should be adjusted according to actual weight.

· **Rocuroniurn:** Despite a lower volume of distribution than in normal-weight subjects, it appears that the pharmacokinetics and pharmacodynamics of rocuronium are comparable in obese and normal-weight subjects. It is therefore preferable to use the ideal weight to calculate the dose of rocuronium. Rocuronium is used in obese patients for rapid sequence induction.

· The recovery time is prolonged if vecuronium is administered per kg of body weight, due to altered hepatic clearance and a greater volume of distribution.

· **Atracuriurn:** No difference was found in volume of distribution, clearance or elimination half-life. It is recommended in cases of renal insufficiency associated with obesity, and the dose is adapted to ideal body weight.

7- Opiates :

· **Fentanyl:** its distribution is not particularly high in obese patients. It can be used and the dose adapted to the ideal weight.

· **Sufentanil**: its volume of distribution is increased but not significantly and its dose is calculated according to corrected weight.

The morphinomimetic which currently offers the most advantages for anaesthesia of the obese seems to be remifentanil, due to its pharmacological properties: small volume of distribution, high clearance, absence of residual effects, particularly respiratory effects, it should be prescribed according to the usual regimens and depending on ideal weight.

8- Inhaled anaesthetic agents :

· **Nitrous oxide:** There is very little data on the use ofnitrous oxide in obese patients. The only obvious disadvantage is a reduction in the fraction of oxygen inspired in these patients, who are at increased risk of hypoxaemia.

· **Halogens:** Fat-soluble halogenated anaesthetics tend toaccumulate in adipose tissue, and the amount administered increases with body weight for the same pharmacological effect.

Sevoflurane, which is less liposoluble than **isoflurane, is associated with an** increase in plasma fluoride concentrations when administered for longer periods. The accumulation of fat-soluble halogens can also lead to delayed awakenings in this population, so the use of **desflurane, which is** less fat-soluble and less

metabolised, seems a logical option.
Overall, **sevoflurane** and **desflurane** are the volatile agents of choice in obese patients.

2.4.2. Sellick manoeuvre :

It consists of exerting pressure vertically. This prevents gastric contents from regurgitating into the pharynx by maintaining oesophageal pressure higher than stomach pressure. Although advocated in most international recommendations, the effectiveness of the Sellick manoeuvre remains controversial insofar as it can make tracheal intubation more difficult for the anaesthetist and be a source of traumatic complications, or even paradoxically encourage regurgitation of gastric contents (see appendix 9).

2.4.3. Rapid sequence induction:

The aim of rapid sequence induction is to achieve rapid intubation in order to avoid hypoxia and inhalation.

2.5. Intubation :

2.5.1. Exposure enhancement manoeuvre :

- **Pressure on the thyroid cartilage, BURP**:

The BURP manoeuvre uses anteroposterior pressure with traction on the top and right of the thyroid cartilage to improve exposure of the glottis.

- **Jackson's improved position:**

This involves placing the external orifice of the auditory canal and the sternal manubrium on a horizontal line. This aligns the buccal, pharyngeal and laryngeal axes to improve exposure of the larynx during intubation. This involves raising the patient's head by around 5 cm, using a cushion (or folded drapes). Anterior flexion of the neck on the thorax aligns the pharyngeal and laryngeal axes, while extension of the head on the neck aligns the buccal axis with the pharyngolaryngeal axis. The combination of these movements exposes the larynx. A similar position can be obtained by "breaking" the pro-tendency table at the headrest (see appendix 10).

2.5.2. Difficult intubation :

A difficult intubation (DI) requires more than two laryngoscopies and/or the use of an alternative technique after optimisation of the head position, with or without external laryngeal manipulation.

• **Equipment for difficult intubation :**

The difficult intubation tray must be part of the operating theatre checklist. The advent of video laryngoscopy in recent years and its development has added to the algorithm for managing difficult intubation in the operating theatre, although it should be pointed out that the use of fibroscopy and video laryngoscopy requires an experienced hand.

• **retrograde intubation :**

Is a technique for oxygenation and intubation in the event of difficult orotracheal or nasotracheal intubation. Cervical ultrasound in the operating theatre has made it easier to perform this technique, and consequently reduced the complications associated with its use.

• **Tracheostomy:** rare in cases where other techniques have failed.

2.7. Maintenance of anaesthesia :

Short-acting anaesthetic agents should be used to maintain anaesthesia.
In addition, monitoring the depth of anaesthesia helps to limit anaesthetic doses and the depth of neuromuscular block.

🕓 **For halogens:** The use of **desflurane**, the least liposoluble and the least metabolised. **Sevoflurane** can also be used.

🕓 **Propofol** used mainly in AIVOC mode.

🕓 The pharmacological properties of remifentanil and **sufentanil** make them te agents of choice for the maintenance of analgesia in morbidly obese patients. They are ideally administered as goal-directed intravenous anaesthesia.

🕓 **For curares:** If muscle relaxation is necessary, only **atracuriurn** and **cisatracuriurn** have slightly altered kinetics in obese patients when administered according to ideal weight. Their maintenance should be titrated and monitored systematically.

2.8. Intraoperative ventilation :

In obese patients, lung and chest wall compliance are reduced, airway resistance is increased, expiratory reserve volume is low and functional residual capacity is reduced, all of which is exacerbated by the supine position. Given the respiratory changes induced by anaesthesia and muscle relaxation, and the risk of perioperative atelectasis, the main objective of intraoperative ventilation in obese patients is to keep the lung "open" during the operation. Respiratory cycle. For this reason, a PEEP of 6 to 10 is recommended for obese patients, depending on their haemodynamics.

Recommended mode of ventilation :

In practice, it is advisable to use the ventilatory mode that you are used to in daily practice, i.e. the one that the team is most familiar with and that it considers to be the safest. The ventilatory mode most often used is the volume-controlled mode. The pressure-controlled mode is recommended by some teams, particularly during laparoscopy, as the decelerating flow rate improves the distribution of airflow in the alveoli. However, studies comparing the two ventilation modes report contradictory data as to the superiority of one mode over the other.

3. The postoperative phase :

3.1. Awakening and extubation :

After assessment of the Aldret score, extubation is envisaged in the proclivity position in the operating theatre or in the post-operative monitoring room.
Prolonged ventilation should be avoided in obese patients, given the high risk of respiratory complications.

3.2. Neuromuscular antagonising agents :

The use of antagonisation at the end of the operation will have a broad indication. Curares are water-soluble agents. However, the vascular sector and extracellular compartments are increased in obese subjects, and if sugammadex is used to decurarise, a dose of 2 mg.kg-1 of ideal weight plus 40% seems optimal.

3.3. Analgesia :

Postoperative multimodal intravenous analgesia should be started intraoperatively. Morphine administration should be cautious. Concomitant oxygen administration is mandatory.

3.4. Thromboprophylaxis :

The prevention of thromboembolic complications must continue in the postoperative period, as must preventive measures such as mobilisation and early postoperative lifting. The doses of drugs used for thromboprophylaxis are adapted to weight and BMI.

3.5. Biological monitoring :

- Renal function after major abdominal surgery (abdominal compartment syndrome)
- CPK (rhabdomyolysis)
- Troponin (increased coronary risk in obese patients).

3.6. Post-operative monitoring :

Post-operative management of obese patients requires prolonged monitoring in the intensive care unit, in view of the specific complications associated with being overweight. In addition to the usual monitoring, surveillance of the obese requires knowledge of the complications specific to this population and the methods for preventing and managing them.

4. Main postoperative complications:

4.1. Respiratory complications :

- In the absence of curarisation monitoring, residual curarisation is a frequent complication in the immediate postoperative period and is responsible for reintubation, which can increase the morbidity and mortality rate.
- Post-operative pulmonary complications are more frequent in obese patients The reduction in ventilatory performance lasts longer after laparotomy in obese patients than in normal-weight patients.
- Post-operative hypoxaemia is common.

• Acute upper airway obstruction is more common in patients with sleep apnoea syndrome, and it is essential to resume assisted ventilation as soon as the patient wakes up.

Prevention :

• It is important to keep obese patients in a semi-seated position from the moment they wake up, and not to extubate them until they are fully awake.

• Respiratory physiotherapy should be as intensive as possible.

4.2. Thromboembolic complications :

The incidence of deep vein thrombosis and pulmonary embolism is higher in the postoperative period, due to venous stasis in the inferior vena cava as a result of immobility, high abdominal pressure, polycythemia, increased inflammatory factors, reduced fibrinolytic activity and endothelial dysfunction.
Prevention is based on thromboprophylactic measures during and after the operation.

4.3. Cardiovascular complications :

Coronary artery disease is a frequent complication in obese patients after an operation, mainly due to the postoperative condition, which aggravates the borderline cardiac condition in obese patients: hypovolaemia, hypoxia, acute anaemia and postoperative pain. The interest of a good postoperative monitoring is the prevention of its occurrence. Other cardiovascular complications can occur postoperatively, in particular rhythm disorders, cardiogenic shock, etc.

4.4. Surgical site complications :

Longer incisions, longer operating times, greater tissue trauma resulting from excessive traction, reduced resistance of adipose tissue and regional defects in oxygenation and vascularisation all contribute to delayed healing and surgical site infections in obese patients.

5. CLINICAL CASE STUDY :

PRE-OPERATIVE STAGE:

5.1.Case presentation :

Mrs D.K, aged 41, married, from and living in RELIZANE, mother of 3 children, weighing 110 kg for a height of 165 cm; with a history of hypothyroidism under treatment for a year and unmonitored arterial hypertension, admitted to the general surgery department of the CHU MOSTAGANEM for scheduled thyroidectomy surgery.

5.2.The History of Illness :

One year ago the patient presented with a visible swelling in the anterior neck. Investigation revealed hypothyroidism with a micronodular thyroid without adenopathy on ultrasound. An indication for thyroidectomy was given, and the patient was referred to us for an anaesthetic consultation.

5.3.Anaesthetic consultation :

5.3.1. Questioning :

• Personal history: allergy to dust.

• Medical :

-Hypothyroidism on levothyrox 150mg for 1 year.

-Hypertension not monitored.

-Functional colonopathy with a tendency to constipation.

-Notion of allergy: allergy to dust without treatment.

• surgery: appendectomy 17 years ago under general anaesthetic with no complications.

• obstetrical: a caesarean section 8 years ago under ALR without complications.

• Family history: RAS

5.3.2. Renorphological data :

• Gender: female

• Age: 41

• Weight 110 kg, height 1.65m

• BMI: 40.4 kg/m2 (morbid obesity).

• ideal weight: = (165) - 100 - ((165 - 150) /2.5) = 57.5 kg

• adjusted weight = (57.5) + 0.4 (110- 57.5)=78. 4 kg

5.3.3. Assessment of respiratory function :

Eupneic patient with good thoracic ampliation, no deformity of the thoracic cage, vesicular murmur clearly perceptible in both lung fields and absence of bronchial rales No underlying respiratory pathology

- Respiratory rate: 12 cycles/min.

- SPO2: 97

- Stop bang calculation: The score is 4 pts

snoring	0 "pt"
daytime fatigue	1 "pt
apnoeas observed by the spouse at night	0 "pt"
HTA	1 "pt
BMI (>35kg/m2)	1 "pt
Age (>50 years)	0 "pt"
neck size > 40cm	1 "pt
Male gender	0 "pt"

Severe risk of OSA stop bang >2 associated with BMI >35

5.3.4. Cardiovascular assessment :

• Absence of signs of heart failure

• Regular heart rate; absence of murmurs; peripheral pulse present and symmetrical. Heart rate 89 bpm, blood pressure 140/70 mmHg.

• absence of varicose veins in the lower limbs

• Venous capital: difficult venous access (veins not visible).

5.3.5. Digestive assessment :

• large, bloated abdomen,

• absence of collateral circulation

• Slow abdominal transit

• The patient's Apfel score is 61%.

	Yes	no	points
Female sex	1		1
Smoking	0	1	1
History of transport	1	0	1
Post-operative morphine	1	0	0
Apfel score	3points = 61		

5.3.6. Renetabolic assessment :

• Morbid obesity with a BMI of 40.4 kg/m2

• No signs of diabetes.

5.3.7. Upper airway exarnen :

✓ search for criteria for difficult intubation :

• BMI 40 kg/m2

• Short neck

• Mallampatie 2

• Flexible and mobile cervical spine.

• Mouth opening greater than 3.5 cm.

• No dentures.

• Thyro-chin distance less than 6.5cm.
✓ search for difficult mask ventilation criteria :
• BMI at 40 kg/m2

• No mandibular or dental pathology

• No snoring

• Severe risk of OSA stop bang >2 associated with BMI >35

Conclusion: Provide ventilation and difficult intubation.

5.3.8. The Exarnens para-clinic :

❖ **Les Exarnens Biologiques :**

• Blood grouping: O positive

• Blood-formula count :

-White blood cells: 6.34x103/mm3

-Red blood cells: 5.40x106/mm3

-Haemoglobin level: 12.3 g/dl

-Haematocrit: 41.4

-CCMH: 32.1g/dl

-Lymphocytes: 2, 68x10 3 /mm3 (42.3%)

-monocytes: 0.49x103/mm3 (7.7%)

-Platelets: 264x 10 3 /mm3 Interpretation: No abnormality.
❖ Haemostasis test: correct

• TP: 100%.

• TCK: 9.80 sec (control 11.00 sec)

❖ Biochemical tests:

• Blood glucose: 1.08 g/1 (normal fasting)

• Urea: 0.26 g/I (normal)

• Creatinemia: 05mg/1(normal)

• Blood calcium: 85.00mg/l (lower limit)

• Phosphorus: 33.00 mg/l (normal)

❖ Hormone tests :

• TSH: 8.1µUI/ml (increased)

• FT3: 4,090 pmol/l (normal)

• FT4:19.94 pmol/l (normal)

❖ Cytopuncture: Cytology suspicious, Bethesda class IV, to be checked by histology.

5.3.9. Radiological Exarnens :

❖ frontal chest X-ray: no tracheal deviation; no pathological parenchymal or pleural images; normal cardiac silhouette.

❖ ECG: regular sinus rhythm at 72/min, no repolarisation disorders, no signs of ventricular overload.

❖ Cervical ultrasound: right cento-lobular thyroid micro-nodule, classified EU-TIRADS 4, on a thyroid gland with a slightly altered echostructure, dysthyroidism, probably inflammatory.

Absence of adenopathy along the vascular axes.

❖ Cardiac ultrasound :

- Non-dilated, non-hypertrophied LV.
- Good segmental and global kinetics.
- Good systolic function.
- LV filling pressure not high.
- Normal-sized OG.
- No significant mitral or aortic valve disease.
- Non-dilated right chambers, good LV systolic function.
- No PAH.

❖ Nasofibroscopy: nasal cavities free. Vocal cords normal in appearance and mobility.

5.4. Assessment of perioperative risks and problems :

5.4.1. Problems posed by the patient : Respiratory :

✓ BMI: 40.4 kg/m2 is morbid obesity

✓ Decreased CRF, diaphragmatic compression

➡ Perioperative hypoxaemia due to respiratory changes associated with obesity

Cardiovascular :

✓ Hypertension: spike in blood pressure

✓ perioperative rhythm disorder

✓ acute coronary syndrome

✓ Increased risk of thromboembolic disease in obese people

✓ Risk of post-operative neuropathy and rhabdomyolysis due to soft tissue compression.

Other problems :

✓ Increased risk of dyslipidaemia BMI > 21kg/m2.

✓ Risk of slow and poor healing of the surgical wound.

5.4.2. Risks associated with anaesthesia :

-Airway management and ventilation

✓ Difficulty of mask ventilation (the presence of a single criterion for difficult mask ventilation).

✓ Risk of difficult intubation

✓ No reserve and risk of rapid desaturation (reduced functional residual capacity and increased oxygen consumption).

✓ Risk of complications on induction, in particular bronchospasm **Risk of full estornac :**

✓ Post-operative digestive disorders: nausea, vomiting and transit disorders very common in obese patients.

✓ Increased risk of inhalation after anaesthetic induction.

Changes in the pharmacokinetics of drugs :

✓ Risk of hypersensitivity to anaesthetic drugs.

✓ Risk of using high doses given the liposolubility of the anaesthetic products used.

✓ Increased elimination of anaesthetic drugs.

✓ Risk of delayed awakening: incorrect dosage of anaesthetic agents. And increased concentrations of alpha 1 acid glycoproteins, hence the notion of residual anaesthesia.

✓ Risk of fat-soluble anaesthetics being released.

✓ Haemodynamic instability related to increased volume of distribution and liposolubility of anaesthetic drugs.

Postoperative problems:

✓ The use of morphine increases the risk of postoperative nausea and vomiting.

5.4.3. Risks associated with surgery :

✓ Intraoperative haemorrhage risk due to injury to cervical vessels, particularly in the case of jugulocarotid curage.

✓ Risk of recurrent and upper laryngeal nerve paralysis.

✓ PONV in the intensive care unit: head extension is one of the factors contributing to PONV.

✓ Hypocalcaemia: in cases of total or subtotal thyroidectomy.

5.4.4. Installation risks :

The head is placed in hyper-extension in a strictly sagittal position, possibly maintained by a headband and an adhesive bandage, which helps to reduce post-operative neck pain.

✓ The arms are held at the sides of the body, while the table is placed in a proclivity position of around 25° to encourage venous drainage of the thyroid gland, but this can lead to a drop in venous return and cardiac output.

✓ Difficulty accessing the patient's head and the peripheral venous line.

✓ postoperative compression neuropathy or rhabdomyolysis.

🕒 **In total :**

Mrs D.K, 41 years old, hypertensive, with a BMI of 40 kg/cm2 who is about to undergo a thyroidectomy. The preoperative work-up is without any particular anomaly, patient classified ASA3, plan for difficult intubation.

5.5.Choice of anaesthetic technique :

For thyroidectomy, general anaesthesia is the technique of choice. It may be combined with a superficial cervical plexus block to improve perioperative analgesia. The patient was scheduled for thyroidectomy under general anaesthetic.

5.6. Inform the patient:

During the anaesthetic consultation, in the presence of the intensive care unit, the anaesthetist and the surgical team, the patient must be informed of the different stages of her treatment, its approximate duration, as well as the possible risk of perioperative complications inherent in the anaesthetic, the surgical procedure, but above all in relation to her high blood pressure and obesity. Information helps to reduce the patient's level of anxiety and encourages cooperation throughout the procedure.

5.7. Preparing the patient :

✓ Weight loss is recommended in order to improve perioperative conditions, but in this case this measure cannot be respected because of the urgent nature of the surgical pathology.
✓ Premedication :

Euthyroidism is essential for patients undergoing thyroidectomy. The aim of medical preparation for the operation is to slow down hormone production or at least to reduce the central and peripheral effects of thyroid hormones.
Prevention of nausea and vomiting.
✓ Rinse: 2 hours for clear liquids, 6 hours for a light meal and at least 8 hours for a full meal.

6. Intraoperative stage :

6.1. Preparation of the operating theatre :

• Checking the patient's file, identity, age, preoperative check-up and anaesthesia record.

• Checking the checklist

• Checking the respirator and gases

• Checking the suction circuit

• Preparation Difficult intubation tray

• Preparing the mattress and heating blanket

• Checking compliance with pre-operative fasting requirements

6.2.Installation and monitoring :

The patient is positioned in the supine position, with the head in a proclivity position (approximately 25°), covered by a heated blanket.
✓ Non-invasive monitoring :

• Electrocardioscope with ST segment analysis

• Non-invasive blood pressure (NIBP), Ill-fitting blood pressure cuff on right arm

• SPO2 pulse oximeter

• Capnography

• Monitoring curarisation

• The parameters at the time of installation are :

-BP =150/75mmhg

- HR=100 beats/min

- FR=12cycle/min

- SP02=99

✓ venous access at 08:38 min:
Difficult approach: after several attempts, a VVP was taken in the left elbow (20G), and an extension tube was fitted to allow injections to be made outside the operating field.
Low-flow isotonic saline.

6.3.Preaching:

• Antibiotic prophylaxis 2 g cefazolin 30 min before induction

• Prevention of nausea and vomiting with dexamethasone 8 mg.

6.4.Pre-oxygenation: starts at 8.45am

Pre-oxygenation for 05 minutes with Fi02 equal to 1 and PEEP 5mmhg

6.5.Induction for general anaesthesia at 8.50 am:

• In the presence of two anaesthetists.

• Rapid sequence induction (narco-analgesia -curare).

• Sellick manoeuvre.

• Anaesthetic drugs :

- Propofol 3mg/kg (3mg*57.5kg=173mg)

- Fentanyl 3µg/kg (3µg *57.5kg =173 µg)

- Rocuronium 0.6mg/kg (0.6mg *57.5kg =35 mg)

• blood pressure: 110/50mmhg

• Manual mask ventilation with Guedel cannula in place.

6.6.Dntubation at 08:54 rnin :

• Exposure to laryngoscopy Cormack 4

• We tried to improve with the BURP manoeuvre but still cormack4

• Two failed attempts at blind intubation, the second using the Bousignac candle

• the patient desaturated 90% of the time

• the patient was treated again with a face mask until saturation reached 100%.

• Intubation using the Bougie de Boussignac with a N°7.5 intubation probe

• Manual ventilation and pulmonary auscultation after balloon inflation: airflow was bilaterally symmetrical in both lung fields

• securing the probe with plasters and gas tape

• Placement of Guedel's cannula

• Installation of an antibacterial filter on the ventilation circuit.

• Patient connected to anaesthesia machine and capnograph at 08:59.

• Re auscultation of both lung fields with good passage of ventilated air, symmetrical and bilateral

• Closure and eye protection

• Placement of a nasogastric tube.

• setting up a bladder catheterisation.

6.7.Ventilatory pararneters :

• Volume-controlled ventilation, semi-closed circuit, VT 460 ml.

• FR at 12/min to be adjusted according to EtCO2

• Inspiratory time over expiratory time 1/2.

• PEEP at 10 cm of H2O and depending on the patient's haemodynamics

• Ventilation with a 50/50 O2/N2O mixture.

• Maximum pressure: 38 mm hg.

6.8.Move into surgical position at 09h 01rnin :

• The head is placed in hyper-extension in a strictly sagittal position, possibly held by an adhesive strip.

• Placement of a block at the tip of the scapula.

• always check the intubation probe at the time of installation.

6.9.Decision at 09:08:

• Blood pressure: 100/50 mmhg

• Heart rate: 85 beats/min.

• Spo2 :100%.

6.10.Maintenance of anaesthesia :

• Maintenance using : Sevoflurane at a concentration of 2.5% combined with boluses of propofol.

• Fentanyl bolus of 50 µg the patient required 3 boluses during the operation.

6.11.Intraoperative monitoring :

• Several bouts of tachycardia were reported, with blood pressure peaks that stabilised after the anaesthetic was deepened.

• An increase in ventilatory pressures of around 38mmhg was observed at 50 minutes after induction, coinciding with a tachycardia and blood pressure spike that resolved with the deepening of the anaesthesia.

• No problems with the capnograph (normocapnia at 36mmhg)

• Absence of intraoperative hypoxia.

Thyroidectomy performed without surgical incident

7. Awakening and extubation :

✓ Administration of 1g paracetmol + parecoxib (sodium) 40 mg IVL

✓ Stop using sevoflurane and nitrous oxide and reset the FiO2 to 100% in the open circuit.

✓ Put the table back in the Trendelenburg position.

✓ Aspiration of gastric contents and removal of the gastric tube at the end of the procedure, followed by careful oral suctioning.

✓ The patient is normothermic.

✓ PEEP always maintained until extubation.

❖ Signs of waking up at 10.45am:

✓ Hemodynamically stable with HR 98 beats/min, BP: 160/08 mmhg

✓ Resumption of spontaneous ventilation; VT mobilisation =405 ml, FR=14 cycles/min, SPO2 =97% on room air

✓ Recovery of laryngeal reflexes, complete decurarisation.

✓ A good way to regain consciousness.

✓ Opening the eyes.

❖ extubation on the operating table at 10.59am: uneventful

8. Postoperative stage :

✓ Patient transferred to post-operative monitoring room

✓ Her haemodynamic parameters remained good:

-BP: 140/80mmhg

- HR: 88 beats/min
- FR: 12 cycles/min

- SPO2:100%

  -T°: 36.8°C

- Correct diuresis
- 3-point VAS pain assessment scale

✓ No incidents were reported.

✓ Her post-intervention treatment file contained.

- Enoxaparin 0.4 ml SC /D until ambulation.
- Omeprazol 40mg/d IVl/d (received).
- Cefazolin 1g IV/6h for 24h (received).
- paracetamol 1g IVL / 6h for 48h received.
- parecoxib (sodium) 40 mg /12 h IVL.

• Basic ration of hydration and electrolytes. A phosphocalcium assessment was requested. Good clinical course with good surgical follow-up.

GENERAL CONCLUSION

Anaesthesia for obese patients is therefore a real challenge for the anaesthesia team, who must provide high-quality care to ensure uncomplicated post-operative recovery. This requires a trained and motivated care team.

BIBLIOGRAPHY

❖ **The books :**

1. J.-E. Bazin, P. Coriat, editor: Arnette. Anaesthesia and resuscitation of the obese patient. Management, prevention of complications and surgery.
2. Xavier Sauvageon, Pierre Viard, Jean-Pierre Tourtier. Anaesthesia products.
3. 41 obesity, OSAS and anaesthesia L. Portmann, E. Albrecht. Manuel pratique d'anesthésie.
4. Bernard DALENS. Traité d'anesthésie générale, published by Arnette.
5. MAPAR. Protocols 2022. Bicêtre Department of Anaesthesia and Intensive Care, 16th edition.
6. Le Guide de l'infirmier anesthésiste editions 2013. Pages (291-292-293)

❖ **Scientific articles :**

1. Audrey De Jong, Daniel Verzilli, Yvan Pouzeratte, Alice Millot, Michaela Penné, Gérald Chanques, Samir Jaber, PhyMedExp, University of Montpellier, INSERM, CNRS, CHU Montpellier ; Département d'Anesthésie-Réanimation, Hôpital Saint-Eloi, 80 avenue Augustin Fliche, 34295 Montpellier cedex, France. SFAR - The Essential Conference 2018 - SFAR. Anaesthesia-resuscitation of the severely obese.
2. S. Valette, R. Cohendy. Anaesthesia and obesity -2008 Département Urgences- Réanimation, CHU de Nîmes, 30029 Nîmes Cedex 9.
3. Pr. Gilles Dhonneur. Hôpitaux Universitaires- Paris Seine -St- Denis Faculté de Médecine Paris 13 Autour de l'Obèse Gestion des Médicaments.
4. G. Lebuffe, G. Andrieu, F. Wierre, K. Gorski, V. Sanders, N. Chalons, B. Vallet. Anaesthesia in the obese overpanel. Anesthesia in the obese overpanel.
5. Dominique SERGENT, Laurent GUIGNARD, Tony JOUIN. THE CONSTRAINTS OF ANAESTHESIA IN GENERAL SURGERY ON OBESE PATIENTS.
6. I. AISSA, F. CLERGUE. Hôpital Tenon, Paris, Hôpital Cantonal Universitaire de Genève.anaesthesia of the obese patient: cardiac and respiratory problems
7. M Carles, M Raucoules-Aimé Pôle d'Anesthésie Réanimations CHU de Nice. Anaesthetic pharmacology of the obese subject.
8. Dr AF DALMAS-LAURENT JLAR 2011. SPECIFIC SOLUTIONS FOR ANAESTHESIA IN THE MORBIDLY OBESE.

9. Dr Audrey, DE JONG Department of Anaesthesia and Intensive Care, Pr Samir Jaber. Peri-operative management of obese patients. Multidisciplinary centre for the management of obesity, Pr David Nocca CHU Montpellier.
10. Ben Souissi Asma Service d'Anesthésie-Réanimation-SMUR CHU Mongi Slim La Marsa, Tunisia. Preoperative evaluation of obese patients.
11. J.E. Bazin, J.M. Constantin, G. Gindre, C. Frey Département d'anesthieréanimation, Hôtel-Dieu, centre hospitalier universitaire, BP 69, 63003 Clermont-Ferrand cedex, Anaesthesia in obese patients.
12. Dr Khalil Tarmiz. Collège national d'anesthésie-réanimation 2007-2008. Anaesthetic management of the obese patient.

13. Audrey de Jong, D. Verzilli, Gerald Chanques, E. Futier, Samir Jaber. Preoperative risk and perioperative management of obese patients.
14. Jean-Étienne Bazin, Director of Research; Pierre Coriat, Director of Research Philippe Juvin. Anaesthesia and resuscitation of the obese patient: management, prevention of complications and surgery.
15. Anaesthesia for obese patients. Dr Olivier PERUS, PH PAR Hôpital Archet 2.

Dr Mehdi Smati. Anaesthetist-resuscitator, Montreuil Hospital. Management of obese patients in anaesthesia.

❖ **Websites :**

• http://www.cfcopies.com/V2/leg/leg_droi.php

• http://www.culture.gouv.fr/culture/infos-pratiques/droits/protection.htm

• https://serval.unil.ch/resource/serval:BIB_07DB168AF17D.P001/REF

• https://www.nysora.com/fr/anesth%C3%A9sie/ob%C3%A9sit%C3%A9/

• https://www.allodocteurs.fr/se-soigner-chirurgie-anesthesie-anesthesie-quelle-prise- encharge-for-obese-persons-19941.html

• https://www.srlf.org/wp-content/uploads/2015/11/20110617-JForm-EmergenciesHonour.pdf

• https://www.decitre.fr/livres/anesthesie-et-reanimation-du-patient-obese-9782718412054.html

• https://www.mapar.org/article/1/Communication%20MAPAR/h1lhsmss/Particul ari
t%25C3%25A9s%20pharmacological%20li%25C3%25A9es%20%25C3%25A0 %20l%25E2%2580%2599ob%25C3%25A9sit%25C3%25A9.pdf

• Website: www.sfar.org

ANNEXES

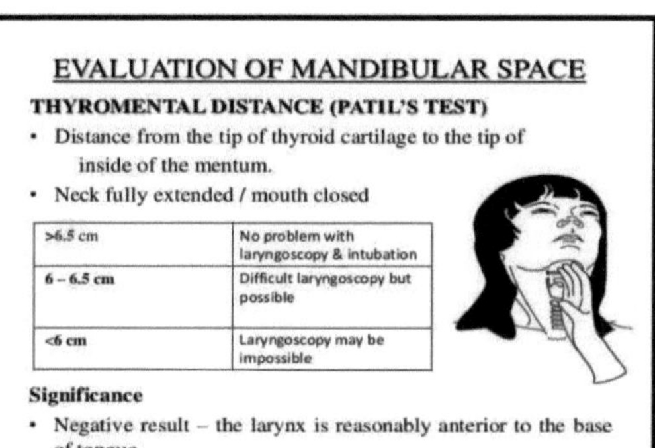

APPENDIX 1 (EVALUATION OF THYROMENTAL

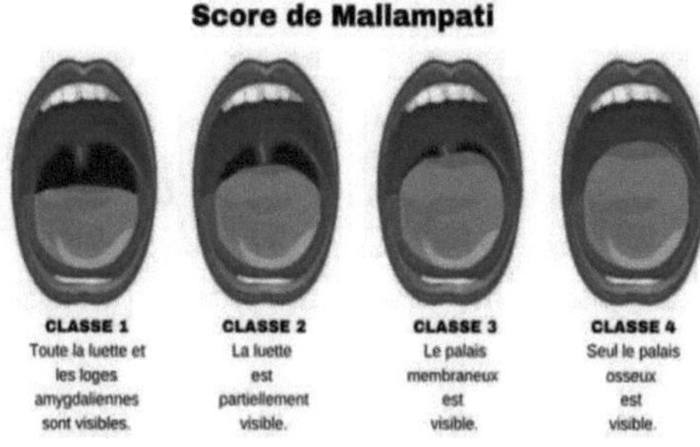

APPENDIX 2 (MALLAMPATIE SCORE)

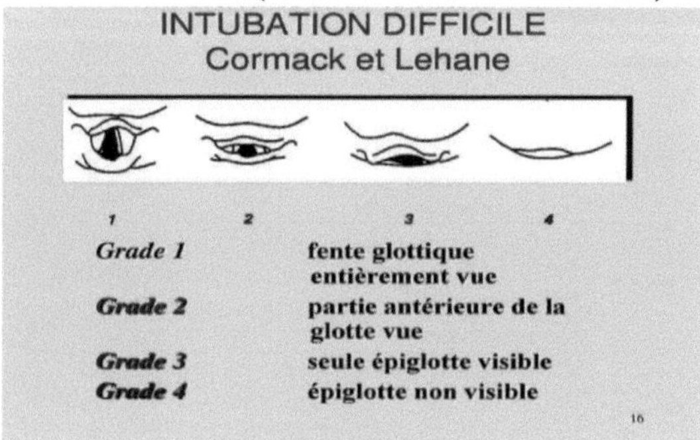

APPENDIX 3

STOP-BANG questionnaire*		
STOP		
S (snore)	Do you *snore* loudly (louder than talking or loud enough to be heard through closed doors)?	Yes/No
T (tired)	Do you often feel *tired*, fatigued, or sleepy during daytime?	Yes/No
O (observed)	Has anyone *observed* you stop breathing during sleep?	Yes/No
P (blood pressure)	Do you have or are you being treated for high blood *pressure*?	Yes/No
BANG		
B (body mass index [BMI])	*BMI* > 35 kg/m²?	Yes/No
A (age)	*Age* > 50 years?	Yes/No
N (neck)	*Neck* circumference > 40 cm?	Yes/No
G (gender)	*Gender* male?	Yes/No

Yes to ≥ 3 questions = high risk of obstructive sleep apnea
Yes to < 3 questions = low risk of obstructive sleep apnea
*Adapted from Chung et al.[20]

• Low risk of SAS if between 0 and 2

• Moderate risk of SAS 3-4

• Severe SAS risk>4 OR stop >=2and BMD >35 OR STOP>=2 and neck circumference >40crn

APPENDIX 4 (STOP-BANG Questionnaire)

Classification de la NYHA	
Classe I	Patient porteur d'une cardiopathie mais sans aucune réduction de l'activité physique.
Classe II	Légère limitation de l'activité physique. Aucune gêne au repos mais l'activité quotidienne ordinaire entraîne une fatigue, une dyspnée ou des palpitations.
Classe III	Limitation marquée des activités physiques. Il n'y a pas de gêne au repos mais une activité moins importante qu'à l'accoutumée provoque des symptômes.
Classe IV	Impossibilité de poursuivre une activité sans gêne : les symptômes de l'insuffisance cardiaque sont présents, même au repos, et la gêne est accrue par toute activité physique.

APPENDIX 5 (NYHA score)

Score de risque cardiaque de Lee		
Calcul du score de Lee classique	Facteur de risque	Calcul du score de Lee clinique
1 point	**Chirurgie à haut risque** définie par une chirurgie vasculaire supra-inguinale, intrathoracique ou intrapéritonéale	
1 point	**Coronaropathie** définie par un antécédent d'infarctus du myocarde, un angor clinique, une utilisation de nitrés, une onde Q sur l'ECG ou un test non invasif de la circulation coronaire positif	1 point
1 point	**Insuffisance cardiaque** définie par un antécédent d'insuffisance cardiaque congestive, d'œdème pulmonaire, une dyspnée nocturne paroxystique, des crépitants bilatéraux ou un galop B3, ou une redistribution vasculaire radiologique	1 point
1 point	**Antécédent d'accident vasculaire cérébral ischémique** ou d'accident cérébral ischémique transitoire	1 point
1 point	**Diabète** avec insulinothérapie	1 point
1 point	**Insuffisance rénale chronique** définie par une créatinine > 2,0 mg/dL (177 µmol/L)	1 point

APPENDIX 6 (LEE score)

	Oui	Non	Score d'Apfel	Risques de NVPO
Sexe féminin	1	0	0	< 10 %
Tabagisme	0	1	1	21 %
Antécédents de NVPO et/ou de mal des transports	1	0	2	39 %
Morphine post-opératoire	1	0	3	61 %
Score d'Apfel	0 à 4		4	79 %

APPENDIX 7 (APFEL SCORE)

Table: Thromboembolic drug prophylaxis in obese patients

Medication	50kg	50a 100kg	100a150kg	Sup150kg
Enoxaparin	20mg1/d	40mg1/d	40mg2/d	60mg2/d
Dalteparine	2500u1/d	5000u1/d	5000u2/d	7500u2/d
Tinzaprine	3500u1/d	4500u1/d	4500u2 /d	6750u2/d

ANNEX 8 (DRUG PROPHYLAXIS)

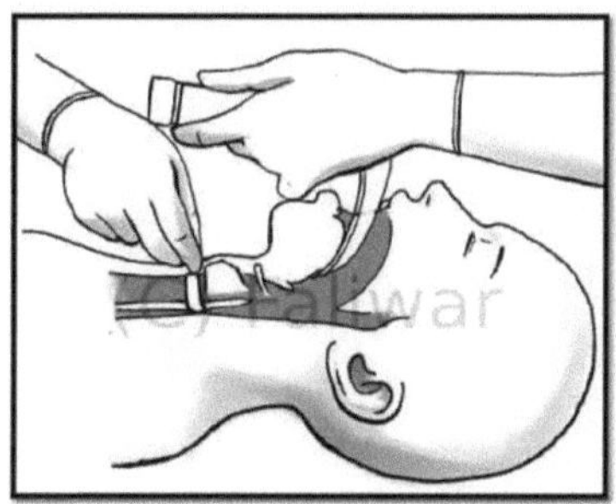

APPENDIX 9 (SELLIK MANOEUVRE)

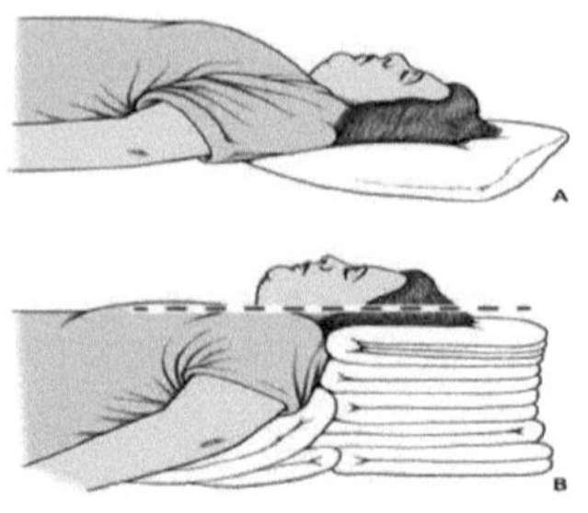

APPENDIX 1O (JACKSON'S POSITION)

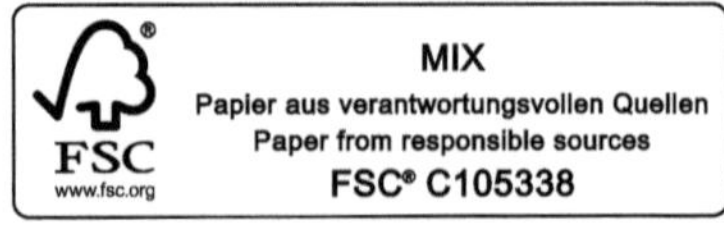

Printed by Books on Demand GmbH, Norderstedt / Germany